Breaking the Mold: Empowering Autistic Adults in the Workplace

Travis Breeding

Copyright © 2023 Travis Breeding

All rights reserved.

ISBN: **9798376311271**

DEDICATION

THIS BOOK IS DEDICATED TO THE MANY IDIVIDUALS IN THE WORLD LIVING WITH ASD AND PEOPLE WHO LOVE AND SUPPORT THEM. I HOPE YOU FIND THIS BOOK USEFUL AND HELPFUL ON YOUR JOURNEY

CONTENTS

	Acknowledgments	i
1	Decoding Diversity: A Guide to Understanding Autism	1
2	Unlocking Potential: Overcoming Workplace Challenges for Autistic Adults	21
3	Hidden Treasures: Discovering the Unique Strengths and Skills of Autistic Adults	42
4	Empowering Differences: Building a Supportive Workplace for Autistic Adults	59
5	Accommodating Abilities: Making Workplace Adjustments for Autistic Adults	78
	About the Author	99

ACKNOWLEDGMENTS

I'd to thank my friends and family for always being here for me and allowing me the time to write. I appreciate all you do for me.

1 DECODING DIVERSITY: A GUIDE TO UNDERSTANDING AUTISM

Autism, also known as Autism Spectrum Disorder (ASD), is a neurodevelopmental disorder that affects how a person communicates and interacts with others. It is a spectrum disorder, meaning that the symptoms and severity of autism can vary greatly from person to person.

The definition of autism has evolved over time, but the current diagnostic criteria for autism are outlined in the Diagnostic and Statistical Manual of Mental Disorders (DSM-5) published by the American

Psychiatric Association. The DSM-5 defines autism as "persistent difficulties in social communication and social interaction across multiple contexts," along with "restricted, repetitive patterns of behavior, interests, or activities."

Symptoms of autism typically become apparent in the first two years of life, although some children may not be diagnosed until later in childhood. The symptoms of autism can include difficulty with social interactions, such as making eye contact or engaging in conversation, repetitive behaviors and routines, difficulty adapting to change, and intense interests in specific topics or objects.

Autism is a complex disorder and its exact cause is not known. Research has suggested that both genetic and environmental factors may play a role in the development of autism. It is important to note that autism is not caused by poor parenting or vaccinations, and is not a result of someone's behavior or personality.

Diagnosis of Autism

Diagnosing autism can be a complex process, and is typically done by a team of professionals that may include a pediatrician, psychologist, or neurologist. The diagnostic process may include a comprehensive evaluation of the individual's development and behavior, as well as input from family members, teachers, and other caregivers.

There is no medical test for autism, but the diagnostic process may include observations of the individual's behavior, communication skills, and social interactions. In addition, standardized developmental assessments may be used to evaluate the individual's language, motor skills, and problem-solving abilities.

It is important to remember that autism is a

spectrum disorder, and the symptoms and severity of autism can vary greatly from person to person. As a result, the diagnostic process is tailored to each individual and may involve multiple evaluations and assessments over time.

Living with Autism

Autism is a lifelong disorder that can have a significant impact on an individual's daily life. However, with early diagnosis and appropriate support, many individuals with autism are able to lead fulfilling and meaningful lives.

Support for individuals with autism can include a combination of therapies and interventions, such as behavioral therapy, speech and language therapy, and occupational therapy. In addition, many individuals with autism benefit from a structured and predictable routine, as well as supportive relationships with family, friends, and caregivers.

It is also important to note that individuals with autism can have a wide range of abilities and talents, and many are able to live independently and pursue careers and interests of their own. With the right support and understanding, individuals with autism can lead fulfilling and meaningful lives.

Autism is a complex and unique disorder that affects how an individual communicates and interacts with others. While it can be challenging for individuals with autism and their families, with the right support and understanding, many individuals with autism are able to lead fulfilling and meaningful lives. It is important to continue to raise awareness about autism and support individuals and families affected by this disorder.

Introduction to Autism in Adults

Autism Spectrum Disorder (ASD) is a neurodevelopmental disorder that affects how a person communicates and interacts with others. While autism is often associated with children, it is a lifelong disorder that affects individuals throughout their lives, including into adulthood.

The prevalence of autism in adults has been the subject of much research in recent years, and the number of adults diagnosed with autism has increased significantly in recent decades. In this ebook, we will examine the current state of research on the prevalence of autism in adult populations, as well as the challenges that adults with autism face and the support and services available to them.

Prevalence of Autism in Adults

The exact prevalence of autism in adult populations is not well understood, as many adults with autism have not been diagnosed or do not receive the support and services they need. However, recent studies have estimated that the prevalence of autism in adults is between 1% and 2% of the general population.

This increase in the number of adults diagnosed with autism is likely due to a combination of factors, including increased awareness of the disorder, improvements in diagnostic tools and practices, and a growing recognition of the needs of adults with autism.

Challenges Faced by Adults with Autism

Adults with autism face a range of challenges in their daily lives, including difficulties with social interactions, communication, and finding and maintaining employment. Many adults with autism also experience mental health concerns, such as anxiety and depression, as well as physical health problems related to their autism.

In addition, many adults with autism have difficulty accessing the support and services they need, including health care, educational opportunities, and employment support. This lack of access to support can have a significant impact on the quality of life of adults with autism, and can make it difficult for them to lead fulfilling and independent lives.

Support and Services for Adults with Autism

Despite the challenges faced by adults with autism, there are a number of support and services available that can help individuals with autism lead fulfilling and meaningful lives. These services can include behavioral and speech therapy, vocational rehabilitation, job training programs, and support groups.

In addition, many states and communities have programs and services specifically designed to support adults with autism, including housing and day programs, vocational training, and social and recreational activities.

The Importance of Diagnosing and Supporting Adults with Autism

Diagnosing and supporting adults with autism is crucial for their well-being and overall quality of life. Early diagnosis can help individuals with autism access the support and services they need to live fulfilling lives, and can also help reduce the risk of co-occurring mental health and physical health problems.

In addition, providing support and services to adults with autism can also help to increase their independence and improve their ability to participate in their communities. This, in turn, can improve their overall quality of life and help to reduce the social and economic costs associated with autism.

Breaking the Mold: Empowering Autistic Adults in the Workplace

The prevalence of autism in adult populations is a growing concern, and there is a need for increased awareness and support for adults with autism. By providing individuals with autism with access to the support and services they need, we can help to improve their quality of life and reduce the social and economic costs associated with autism.

Introduction to Autism and Employment

Autism Spectrum Disorder (ASD) is a neurodevelopmental disorder that affects how a person communicates and interacts with others. While autism is often associated with children, it is a lifelong disorder that affects individuals throughout their lives, including in the workplace.

Employment is an important aspect of adult life for individuals with autism, as it provides a sense of purpose, a sense of accomplishment, and a source of financial stability. In this ebook, we will examine the importance of employment for autistic individuals, and the challenges that individuals with autism face in finding and maintaining employment.

The Benefits of Employment for Autistic Individuals

Employment provides many benefits for individuals with autism, including financial stability, a sense of purpose and accomplishment, and opportunities for social interaction and community engagement. In addition, employment can help to increase individuals' independence and reduce their reliance on caregivers and support services.

For individuals with autism who may struggle with social interactions, employment can also provide a structured and predictable environment where they can focus on their strengths and skills, and build confidence and self-esteem.

The Challenges of Finding and Maintaining Employment for Autistic Individuals

Despite the many benefits of employment for autistic individuals, finding and maintaining employment can be challenging for many individuals with autism. Some of the challenges faced by individuals with autism in the workplace include difficulties with communication, social interactions, and adapting to new and changing environments.

In addition, many employers are not familiar with autism and may not understand the strengths and abilities of individuals with autism, leading to missed opportunities for employment. This lack of understanding and awareness can also result in negative attitudes and stereotypes about individuals with autism, making it even more difficult for them to find and maintain employment.

The Importance of Employer Awareness and Inclusion

To support individuals with autism in finding and maintaining employment, it is important for employers to be aware of autism and to create inclusive workplace environments. Employers can support individuals with autism by providing accommodations and support, and by understanding the unique strengths and abilities of individuals with autism.

In addition, employers can help to raise awareness of autism and to break down negative stereotypes and attitudes by promoting diversity and inclusion in the workplace. This can create a more welcoming and supportive environment for individuals with autism, and help to increase their chances of finding and maintaining employment.

Practical Strategies for Supporting Autistic Individuals in the Workplace

In addition to raising awareness and promoting inclusion, there are a number of practical strategies that employers and coworkers can use to support individuals with autism in the workplace. These strategies can include providing accommodations, such as flexible schedules and modified duties, and providing training and support for coworkers to better understand and support individuals with autism.

In addition, employers can support individuals with autism by providing opportunities for professional development and career advancement, and by creating a welcoming and inclusive workplace culture.

The Role of Vocational Rehabilitation and Support Services

Vocational rehabilitation and support services can also play an important role in helping individuals with autism find and maintain employment. These services can include job training programs, job placement services, and support for individuals with autism in the workplace.

Vocational rehabilitation and support services can help individuals with autism to develop the skills and confidence they need to succeed in the workplace, and to find and maintain employment that is meaningful and fulfilling.

Introduction to Autism and Employment

Autism Spectrum Disorder (ASD) is a neurodevelopmental disorder that affects how a person communicates and interacts with others. While autism is often associated with children, it is a lifelong disorder that affects individuals throughout their lives, including in the workplace.

Employment is an important aspect of adult life for individuals with autism, as it provides a sense of purpose, a sense of accomplishment, and a source of financial stability. In this ebook, we will examine the employment challenges faced by autistic adults, and begin to have a conversation about practical solutions to these challenges.

The Challenges of Finding Employment for Autistic Adults

Finding employment can be a significant challenge for autistic adults. Many employers are not familiar with autism and may not understand the strengths and abilities of individuals with autism, leading to missed opportunities for employment. This lack of understanding and awareness can also result in negative attitudes and stereotypes about individuals with autism, making it even more difficult for them to find employment.

In addition, individuals with autism may face challenges in the job search process, including difficulties with communication, social interactions, and adapting to new and changing environments.

The Challenges of Maintaining Employment for Autistic Adults

Maintaining employment can also be a challenge for autistic adults. Individuals with autism may struggle with communication, social interactions, and adapting to new and changing work environments, leading to difficulties in building relationships with coworkers and supervisors.

In addition, individuals with autism may need accommodations and support to succeed in the workplace, and may face challenges in securing these accommodations. Employers and coworkers may not understand the needs of individuals with autism, leading to difficulties in finding effective solutions to these challenges.

The Importance of Employer Awareness

and Inclusion

To support individuals with autism in finding and maintaining employment, it is important for employers to be aware of autism and to create inclusive workplace environments. Employers can support individuals with autism by providing accommodations and support, and by understanding the unique strengths and abilities of individuals with autism.

In addition, employers can help to raise awareness of autism and to break down negative stereotypes and attitudes by promoting diversity and inclusion in the workplace. This can create a more welcoming and supportive environment for individuals with autism, and help to increase their chances of finding and maintaining employment.

The Role of Vocational Rehabilitation and Support Services

Vocational rehabilitation and support services can also play an important role in helping individuals with autism find and maintain employment. These services can include job training programs, job placement services, and support for individuals with autism in the workplace.

Vocational rehabilitation and support services can help individuals with autism to develop the skills and confidence they need to succeed in the workplace, and to find and maintain employment that is meaningful and fulfilling.

The Importance of Employee Advocacy and Self-Advocacy

In addition to the support of employers, coworkers, and support services, individuals with autism can also play an important role in advocating for themselves in the workplace. This can include speaking up about their needs and seeking accommodations, as well as building relationships with coworkers and supervisors to build a supportive work environment.

Employment is an important aspect of adult life for individuals with autism, providing financial stability, a sense of purpose, and opportunities for social interaction and community engagement. However, finding and maintaining employment can be challenging for individuals with autism, and requires the support of employers, coworkers, and support services.

By raising awareness and promoting inclusion, providing accommodations and support, and advocating for themselves, individuals with autism can succeed in the workplace and build meaningful and fulfilling careers.

2 UNLOCKING POTENTIAL: OVERCOMING WORKPLACE CHALLENGES FOR AUTISTIC ADULTS

Introduction to Autism and Communication in the Workplace

Autism Spectrum Disorder (ASD) is a neurodevelopmental disorder that affects how individuals communicate and interact with others. While autism is often associated with children, it is a lifelong disorder that affects individuals throughout their lives, including in the workplace.

One of the key challenges faced by individuals with autism in the workplace is difficulty with social and communication skills. These difficulties can impact an individual's ability to build relationships with coworkers and supervisors, to effectively communicate their needs and wants, and to succeed in their job.

Understanding Social and Communication Difficulties in Autism

Individuals with autism may experience difficulties with social communication, including nonverbal communication, such as gestures and facial expressions, as well as difficulties with understanding the nuances of social interactions.

In the workplace, these difficulties can impact an individual's ability to build relationships with coworkers and supervisors, leading to feelings of isolation and exclusion. Additionally, individuals with autism may struggle with understanding and communicating their needs and wants, which can lead to misunderstandings and conflicts in the workplace.

The Impact of Social and Communication Difficulties in the Workplace

The impact of social and communication difficulties in the workplace can be significant for individuals with autism. These difficulties can lead to difficulties in building relationships with coworkers and supervisors, as well as difficulties in effectively communicating their needs and wants.

In addition, individuals with autism may struggle with adapting to new and changing work environments, leading to increased stress and anxiety. These difficulties can also impact an individual's job performance and satisfaction, leading to decreased job stability and reduced opportunities for advancement.

Strategies for Overcoming Social and Communication Difficulties in the

Workplace

There are several strategies that individuals with autism, as well as employers and coworkers, can use to overcome social and communication difficulties in the workplace. These strategies include:

Providing accommodations and support, such as visual aids and extra time for processing information

Encouraging and facilitating open communication between individuals with autism and their coworkers and supervisors

Building relationships and establishing support networks in the workplace

Providing training and education for individuals with autism and their coworkers and supervisors on effective communication and social skills

Promoting a culture of inclusiveness and understanding in the workplace

The Importance of Employer Awareness and Inclusion

To support individuals with autism in overcoming social and communication difficulties in the workplace, it is important for employers to be aware of autism and to create inclusive workplace environments. Employers can support individuals with autism by providing accommodations and support, and by understanding the unique strengths and abilities of individuals with autism.

In addition, employers can help to raise awareness of autism and to break down negative stereotypes and attitudes by promoting diversity and inclusion in the workplace. This can create a more welcoming and supportive environment for individuals with autism, and help to reduce the impact of social and communication difficulties in the workplace.

The Role of Vocational Rehabilitation and

Support Services

Vocational rehabilitation and support services can also play an important role in helping individuals with autism overcome social and communication difficulties in the workplace. These services can include job training programs, job placement services, and support for individuals with autism in the workplace.

Vocational rehabilitation and support services can help individuals with autism to develop the skills and confidence they need to succeed in the workplace, and to overcome the challenges of social and communication difficulties in the workplace.

Introduction to Unspoken Rules and Norms in the Workplace

The workplace is full of unspoken rules and norms that can be difficult for anyone to navigate, but particularly challenging for individuals with autism. These unspoken rules and norms can include social expectations, communication styles, and unwritten rules about how work is done.

For individuals with autism, these unspoken rules and norms can be especially challenging because they often rely on social cues and intuition to understand the expectations and norms of a given situation. In the workplace, these skills can be difficult to develop and maintain, leading to misunderstandings and difficulties in adapting to the workplace culture.

The Impact of Unspoken Rules and Norms on Autistic Adults

The difficulties associated with navigating unspoken rules and norms in the workplace can have a significant impact on individuals with autism. These difficulties can lead to misunderstandings and conflicts with coworkers and supervisors, leading to decreased job satisfaction and decreased opportunities for advancement.

In addition, the stress and anxiety associated with navigating unspoken rules and norms in the workplace can also have a negative impact on an individual's mental health and overall well-being. These difficulties can also impact an individual's job performance, leading to decreased job stability and reduced opportunities for advancement.

Understanding Unspoken Rules and Norms in the Workplace

To overcome the difficulties associated with navigating unspoken rules and norms in the workplace, it is important for individuals with autism to understand the expectations and norms of the workplace. This understanding can be achieved through observation and feedback from coworkers and supervisors, as well as through formal training and education on effective communication and social skills.

In addition, individuals with autism can benefit from developing a better understanding of their own strengths and limitations, and using this understanding to better navigate the challenges of the workplace.

Strategies for Navigating Unspoken Rules and Norms in the Workplace

There are several strategies that individuals with autism can use to navigate the challenges of unspoken rules and norms in the workplace. These strategies include:

Building relationships with coworkers and supervisors, and seeking feedback and support when needed

Seeking out training and education on effective communication and social skills

Observing the behavior and communication styles of others in the workplace, and adapting accordingly

Encouraging open and honest communication with coworkers and supervisors about expectations and norms in the workplace

Seeking out support from vocational rehabilitation and support services, if needed

The Importance of Employer Awareness and Inclusion

In order to support individuals with autism in navigating the challenges of unspoken rules and norms in the workplace, it is important for employers to be aware of autism and to create inclusive workplace environments. Employers can support individuals with autism by providing accommodations and support, and by understanding the unique strengths and abilities of individuals with autism.

In addition, employers can help to raise awareness of autism and to break down negative stereotypes and attitudes by promoting diversity and inclusion in the workplace. This can create a more welcoming and supportive environment for individuals with autism, and help to reduce the impact of unspoken rules and norms in the workplace.

The Role of Vocational Rehabilitation and Support Services

Vocational rehabilitation and support services can also play an important role in helping individuals with autism navigate the challenges of unspoken rules and norms in the workplace. These services can include job training programs, job placement services, and support for individuals with autism in the workplace.

Vocational rehabilitation and support services can help individuals with autism to develop the skills and confidence they need to succeed in the workplace, and to navigate the challenges of unspoken rules and norms in the workplace.

Introduction to Sensory Sensitivities and Environmental Considerations in the Workplace

Individuals with autism often experience sensory sensitivities that can impact their ability to function in the workplace. These sensitivities can include sensitivity to light, sound, touch, and other sensory stimuli. These sensitivities can lead to discomfort, stress, and anxiety in the workplace, making it difficult for individuals with autism to perform their job duties effectively.

In addition, the physical environment of the workplace can also impact the well-being and performance of individuals with autism. Factors such as lighting, noise levels, and temperature can all impact an individual's ability to function in the workplace, making it important for employers to consider these factors when creating a supportive work environment for individuals with autism.

Understanding Sensory Sensitivities and Environmental Considerations in the Workplace

To understand the impact of sensory sensitivities and environmental considerations in the workplace, it is important to consider the unique needs and experiences of individuals with autism. For example, individuals with autism may be sensitive to bright or flickering lights, or to high levels of noise, which can impact their ability to focus and concentrate on the job.

It is also important to understand that these sensitivities can vary widely from person to person, and that what works for one individual with autism may not work for another. This means that it is important to work with each individual with autism to understand their specific needs and to accommodate these needs in the workplace.

Strategies for Accommodating Sensory Sensitivities and Environmental Considerations in the Workplace

To accommodate sensory sensitivities and environmental considerations in the workplace, employers can take several steps, including:

Providing adjustable lighting and noise levels in the workplace

Offering flexible work arrangements, such as the option to work from home or to work in a quieter environment

Providing access to sensory tools and equipment, such as noise-cancelling headphones or fidget toys

Encouraging open communication with employees with autism about their needs and concerns

The Importance of Employer Awareness and Inclusion

It is important for employers to be aware of the impact of sensory sensitivities and environmental considerations on individuals with autism, and to take steps to accommodate these needs in the workplace. This can include providing training and education for employees and managers on autism and sensory sensitivities, and promoting diversity and inclusion in the workplace.

In addition, employers can support individuals with autism by providing accommodations and support, and by understanding the unique strengths and abilities of individuals with autism. This can help to reduce the impact of sensory sensitivities and environmental considerations in the workplace, and can lead to improved job satisfaction and performance for individuals with autism.

The Role of Vocational Rehabilitation and Support Services

Vocational rehabilitation and support services can also play an important role in helping individuals with autism navigate the challenges of sensory sensitivities and environmental considerations in the workplace. These services can include job training programs, job placement services, and support for individuals with autism in the workplace.

Vocational rehabilitation and support services can help individuals with autism to develop the skills and confidence they need to succeed in the workplace, and to navigate the challenges of sensory sensitivities and environmental considerations in the workplace.

Conclusion

In conclusion, sensory sensitivities and environmental considerations can have a significant impact on the ability of individuals with autism to function in the workplace. By understanding the unique needs and experiences of individuals with autism, and by taking steps to accommodate these needs in the workplace, employers can create a supportive and inclusive work environment that benefits both employees and the organization as a whole.

Introduction to the Challenge of Change and Unpredictability in the Workplace for Autistic Adults

Individuals with autism often struggle with change and unpredictability in the workplace. This can include changes in routines, work tasks, or the physical environment. The challenges associated with change and unpredictability can lead to stress, anxiety, and decreased job performance for individuals with autism.

Understanding the Impact of Change and Unpredictability in the Workplace

To understand the impact of change and unpredictability in the workplace, it is important to consider the unique perspectives and experiences of individuals with autism. For example, individuals with autism may rely heavily on routine and structure to help them manage their day-to-day lives, and sudden changes in routine can cause significant stress and anxiety.

Additionally, changes in the physical environment, such as a new office layout or a reorganization of the workplace, can be particularly challenging for individuals with autism. This is because individuals with autism may struggle with adapting to new environments, and may have trouble navigating the changes and unpredictability that come with a new workplace setting.

Strategies for Managing Change and Unpredictability in the Workplace

To help individuals with autism manage change and unpredictability in the workplace, employers can take several steps, including:

Providing advanced notice of changes in routine or the physical environment

Offering support and resources, such as counseling or therapy, to help individuals with autism manage stress and anxiety

Encouraging open communication with employees with autism about their needs and concerns

Providing opportunities for employees with autism to practice adapting to change and unpredictability in a safe and supportive environment

The Importance of Employer Awareness and Inclusion

It is important for employers to be aware of the impact of change and unpredictability on individuals with autism, and to take steps to accommodate these needs in the workplace. This can include providing training and education for employees and managers on autism and the challenges associated with change and unpredictability, and promoting diversity and inclusion in the workplace.

In addition, employers can support individuals with autism by providing accommodations and support, and by understanding the unique strengths and abilities of individuals with autism. This can help to reduce the impact of change and unpredictability in the workplace, and can lead to improved job satisfaction and performance for individuals with autism.

The Role of Vocational Rehabilitation and Support Services

Vocational rehabilitation and support services can also play an important role in helping individuals with autism navigate the challenges of change and unpredictability in the workplace. These services can include job training programs, job placement services, and support for individuals with autism in the workplace.

Vocational rehabilitation and support services can help individuals with autism to develop the skills and confidence they need to succeed in the workplace, and to navigate the challenges of change and unpredictability in the workplace.

Conclusion

In conclusion, change and unpredictability in the workplace can pose significant challenges for individuals with autism. By understanding the unique needs and experiences of individuals with autism, and by taking steps to accommodate these needs in the workplace, employers can create a supportive and inclusive work environment that benefits both employees and the organization as a whole.

3 HIDDEN TREASURES: DISCOVERING THE UNIQUE SKILLS AND STRENGTHS OF AUTISTIC ADULTS

Introduction to the Ability of Autistic Individuals to Pay Attention to Detail and Focus on a Task

Individuals with autism often have a strong ability to pay attention to detail and to focus on a task for extended periods of time. This ability can be a significant strength in the workplace, as it can result in high-quality work, improved productivity, and increased job satisfaction for individuals with autism.

Understanding the Attention to Detail and Task Focus of Autistic Individuals

To understand the attention to detail and task focus of individuals with autism, it is important to consider their unique perspectives and experiences. For example, individuals with autism may have an intense focus on a particular task or subject, which can lead to a heightened attention to detail and a deep understanding of the task at hand.

Additionally, individuals with autism may be less prone to distractions and may have a stronger ability to filter out distractions, which can allow them to maintain their focus on a task for extended periods of time.

The Benefits of Autistic Individuals' Ability to Pay Attention to Detail and Focus on a Task

The ability of individuals with autism to pay attention to detail and focus on a task can have several benefits in the workplace, including:

Improved productivity and quality of work

Increased job satisfaction and motivation

Improved accuracy and attention to detail

Ability to complete tasks quickly and efficiently

The Importance of Employer Awareness and Inclusion

It is important for employers to be aware of the strengths and abilities of individuals with autism, including their ability to pay attention to detail and focus on a task. This awareness can lead to improved hiring and workplace practices, and can help to create a supportive and inclusive work environment for individuals with autism.

In addition, employers can support individuals with autism by providing accommodations and support, and by understanding the unique strengths and abilities of individuals with autism. This can help to harness their attention to detail and task focus, and can lead to improved job satisfaction and performance for individuals with autism.

The Role of Vocational Rehabilitation and Support Services

Vocational rehabilitation and support services can also play an important role in helping individuals with autism to maximize their ability to pay attention to detail and focus on a task in the workplace. These services can include job training programs, job placement services, and support for individuals with autism in the workplace.

Vocational rehabilitation and support services can help individuals with autism to develop the skills and confidence they need to succeed in the workplace, and to harness their ability to pay attention to detail and focus on a task.

Conclusion

In conclusion, the ability of individuals with autism to pay attention to detail and focus on a task can be a significant strength in the workplace. By understanding the unique needs and experiences of individuals with autism, and by taking steps to accommodate these needs in the workplace, employers can create a supportive and inclusive work environment that benefits both employees and the organization as a whole.

Introduction to the Strong Work Ethic and Reliability of Autistic Individuals

Individuals with autism are often known for their strong work ethic and reliability in the workplace. This combination of traits can be a valuable asset to employers, and can result in improved job satisfaction and performance for individuals with autism.

Understanding the Strong Work Ethic and Reliability of Autistic Individuals

To understand the strong work ethic and reliability of individuals with autism, it is important to consider their unique perspectives and experiences. For example, individuals with autism may have a strong sense of responsibility and may take their work seriously, which can result in a strong commitment to their job and a dedication to completing tasks to the best of their ability.

Additionally, individuals with autism may have a strong sense of routine and may prefer a structured and predictable work environment, which can result in improved reliability and a consistent work ethic.

The Benefits of Autistic Individuals' Strong Work Ethic and Reliability

The strong work ethic and reliability of individuals with autism can have several benefits in the workplace, including:

Improved job performance and productivity

Increased job satisfaction and motivation

Improved accuracy and attention to detail

Consistent and dependable work behavior

The Importance of Employer Awareness and Inclusion

It is important for employers to be aware of the strengths and abilities of individuals with autism, including their strong work ethic and reliability. This awareness can lead to improved hiring and workplace practices, and can help to create a supportive and inclusive work environment for individuals with autism.

In addition, employers can support individuals with autism by providing accommodations and support, and by understanding the unique strengths and abilities of individuals with autism. This can help to harness their strong work ethic and reliability, and can lead to improved job satisfaction and performance for individuals with autism.

The Role of Vocational Rehabilitation and Support Services

Vocational rehabilitation and support services can also play an important role in helping individuals with autism to maximize their strong work ethic and reliability in the workplace. These services can include job training programs, job placement services, and support for individuals with autism in the workplace.

Vocational rehabilitation and support

services can help individuals with autism to develop the skills and confidence they need to succeed in the workplace, and to harness their strong work ethic and reliability.

Conclusion

In conclusion, the strong work ethic and reliability of individuals with autism can be a significant strength in the workplace. By understanding the unique needs and experiences of individuals with autism, and by taking steps to accommodate these needs in the workplace, employers can create a supportive and inclusive work environment that benefits both employees and the organization as a whole.

Introduction to the Unique Perspectives and Problem-Solving Skills of Autistic Adults

Autistic adults have unique perspectives and problem-solving skills that can bring value to the workplace. Despite the challenges they face, individuals with autism have the ability to bring fresh and innovative ideas to the table, and to approach problems in new and creative ways.

Understanding the Unique Perspectives of Autistic Adults

Individuals with autism may have a different way of perceiving the world, which can result in unique perspectives and insights. For example, individuals with autism may have a strong attention to detail and may be able to see patterns and connections that others may miss.

Additionally, individuals with autism may have a heightened sensitivity to sensory information, which can result in a heightened awareness of their surroundings and an ability to notice things that others may not.

The Benefits of Autistic Adults' Unique

Perspectives

The unique perspectives of autistic adults can bring several benefits to the workplace, including:

Improved problem-solving and creative thinking

Fresh and innovative ideas and approaches

Improved accuracy and attention to detail

Heightened awareness of their surroundings and environment

The Importance of Employer Awareness and Inclusion

It is important for employers to be aware of the strengths and abilities of individuals with autism, including their unique perspectives and problem-solving skills. This awareness can lead to improved hiring and workplace practices, and can help to create a supportive and inclusive work environment for individuals with autism.

In addition, employers can support individuals with autism by providing accommodations and support, and by understanding the unique perspectives and abilities of individuals with autism. This can help to harness their unique perspectives and problem-solving skills, and can lead to improved job satisfaction and performance for individuals with autism.

The Role of Vocational Rehabilitation and Support Services

Vocational rehabilitation and support services can also play an important role in helping individuals with autism to maximize their unique perspectives and problem-solving skills in the workplace. These services can include job training programs, job placement services, and support for individuals with autism in the workplace.

Vocational rehabilitation and support services can help individuals with autism to develop the skills and confidence they need to succeed in the workplace, and to harness their unique perspectives and problem-solving skills.

Conclusion

In conclusion, the unique perspectives and problem-solving skills of individuals with autism can be significant strengths in the workplace. By understanding the unique needs and experiences of individuals with autism, and by taking steps to accommodate these needs in the workplace, employers can create a supportive and inclusive work environment that benefits both employees and the organization as a whole.

Introduction to the Honesty and Integrity of Autistic Adults in the Workplace

Autistic adults are known for their honesty and integrity, which can be valuable assets in the workplace. Despite the challenges they face, individuals with autism have a strong sense of ethics and a commitment to doing the right thing.

Understanding the Honesty and Integrity of Autistic Adults

Individuals with autism often have a strong sense of right and wrong, and are guided by their own personal moral code. They may have a heightened sense of honesty and integrity, and are often straightforward and honest in their interactions with others.

Additionally, individuals with autism may have difficulty understanding or navigating complex social interactions, which can result in a focus on honesty and straightforward communication.

The Benefits of Autistic Adults' Honesty and Integrity

The honesty and integrity of autistic adults can bring several benefits to the workplace, including:

Improved trust and confidence in coworkers and employers

A commitment to ethical behavior and doing the right thing

Improved communication and transparency

A focus on accuracy and attention to detail

The Importance of Employer Awareness and Inclusion

It is important for employers to be aware of the strengths and abilities of individuals with autism, including their honesty and integrity. This awareness can lead to improved hiring and workplace practices, and can help to create a supportive and inclusive work environment for individuals with autism.

In addition, employers can support individuals with autism by providing accommodations and support, and by understanding the unique needs and experiences of individuals with autism. This can help to harness their honesty and integrity, and can lead to improved job satisfaction and performance for individuals with autism.

The Role of Vocational Rehabilitation and Support Services

Vocational rehabilitation and support services can also play an important role in helping individuals with autism to maximize their honesty and integrity in the workplace. These services can include job training programs, job placement services, and support for individuals with autism in the workplace.

Vocational rehabilitation and support services can help individuals with autism to develop the skills and confidence they need to succeed in the workplace, and to harness their honesty and integrity.

Conclusion

In conclusion, the honesty and integrity of individuals with autism can be significant strengths in the workplace. By understanding the unique needs and experiences of individuals with autism, and by taking steps to accommodate these needs in the workplace, employers can create a supportive and inclusive work environment that benefits both employees and the organization as a whole.

4 EMPOWERING DIFFERENCES: BUILDING A SUPPORTIVE WORKPLACE FOR AUTISTIC ADULTS

Introduction to the Importance of Clear Communication and Structure for Autistic Adults in the Workplace

Autistic adults often struggle with social and communication difficulties, making it important for the workplace to provide clear communication and structure to support them in their jobs. This ebook will explore why clear communication and structure are crucial for the success of autistic adults in the workplace, and what can be done to ensure these needs are met.

The Challenges of Communication and Structure in the Workplace for Autistic Adults

Autistic adults often struggle with social and communication difficulties, which can make it challenging for them to navigate the workplace. These challenges may include difficulty understanding nonverbal cues, difficulty with small talk and socializing, and trouble interpreting sarcasm or humor. Additionally, some individuals with autism may struggle with change and unpredictability, making it important for the workplace to provide clear structure and routine.

The Benefits of Clear Communication and Structure

Providing clear communication and structure in the workplace can have several benefits for autistic adults, including:

Improved understanding of job expectations and responsibilities

Reduced stress and anxiety

Improved job satisfaction

Improved job performance

Best Practices for Clear Communication

To support autistic adults in the workplace, it is important to provide clear communication in a way that they can understand. Some best practices for clear communication include:

Using plain and straightforward language

Breaking down complex instructions into smaller, manageable steps

Providing written instructions or visual aids to support understanding

Avoiding sarcasm and humor

Being mindful of nonverbal cues and body

language

Best Practices for Providing Structure and Routine

In addition to clear communication, providing structure and routine in the workplace can also be beneficial for autistic adults. Some best practices for providing structure and routine include:

Creating a consistent schedule and routine

Providing advance warning of changes or disruptions

Using visual aids or timers to support transitions

Providing predictable routines for breaks and lunchtime

The Role of Employers and Coworkers

Employers and coworkers play an important role in supporting autistic adults in the workplace. By being aware of the challenges faced by individuals with autism, and by taking steps to accommodate their needs, employers and coworkers can help to create a supportive and inclusive work environment.

This may include providing accommodations such as flexible schedules or quiet workspaces, and taking steps to ensure that communication is clear and easy to understand. Additionally, employers and coworkers can support individuals with autism by being understanding and patient, and by avoiding behavior that may cause stress or anxiety.

Conclusion

In conclusion, clear communication and structure are crucial for the success of autistic adults in the workplace. By taking steps to accommodate these needs, employers and coworkers can help to create a supportive and inclusive work environment that benefits both employees and the organization as a whole.

Introduction to Providing Accommodations and Modifications for Autistic Adults on the Job

Autistic adults often face unique challenges in the workplace, but with appropriate accommodations and modifications, they can thrive and succeed in their careers. This ebook will explore the importance of providing accommodations and modifications for autistic adults on the job, and will provide practical tips and strategies for doing so.

Understanding the Needs of Autistic Adults in the Workplace

Before making accommodations and modifications for autistic adults in the workplace, it is important to understand their unique needs and challenges. Some common difficulties faced by autistic individuals in the workplace include social and communication difficulties, sensory sensitivities, and difficulty with change and unpredictability.

The Benefits of Providing Accommodations and Modifications

Providing accommodations and modifications in the workplace can have several benefits for autistic adults, including:

Improved job performance

Increased job satisfaction

Reduced stress and anxiety

Improved overall wellbeing

Best Practices for Providing Accommodations

There are many accommodations that can be made to support autistic adults in the workplace. Some best practices for providing accommodations include:

Allowing for flexible schedules or quiet workspaces

Providing visual aids or timers to support transitions

Offering accommodations for sensory sensitivities, such as noise-cancelling headphones or special lighting

Providing support and resources for social and communication difficulties

Best Practices for Providing Modifications

In addition to accommodations, modifications can also be made to support autistic adults in the workplace. Some best practices for providing modifications include:

Breaking down complex instructions into smaller, manageable steps

Providing clear and straightforward

instructions

Allowing for additional time and support for task completion

Providing a quiet and distraction-free workspace

The Role of Employers and Coworkers

Employers and coworkers play an important role in supporting autistic adults in the workplace. By being aware of the needs of individuals with autism and making appropriate accommodations and modifications, employers and coworkers can help to create a supportive and inclusive work environment.

This may include providing accommodations such as flexible schedules or quiet workspaces, and taking steps to ensure that communication is clear and easy to understand. Additionally, employers and coworkers can support individuals with autism by being understanding and patient, and by avoiding behavior that may cause stress or anxiety.

Conclusion

In conclusion, providing accommodations and modifications in the workplace is crucial for the success of autistic adults. By understanding the unique needs and challenges faced by individuals with autism, and by making appropriate accommodations and modifications, employers and coworkers can help to create a supportive and inclusive work environment that benefits both employees and the organization as a whole.

Introduction to Creating a Safe and Inclusive Work Environment for Autistic Adults

Autistic adults face unique challenges in the workplace, and it is essential to create a safe and inclusive work environment that supports and accommodates their needs.

This ebook will explore the importance of creating a safe and inclusive work environment for autistic adults, and will provide practical tips and strategies for doing so.

Understanding the Needs of Autistic Adults in the Workplace

Before creating a safe and inclusive work environment for autistic adults, it is important to understand their unique needs and challenges. Some common difficulties faced by autistic individuals in the workplace include social and communication difficulties, sensory sensitivities, and difficulty with change and unpredictability.

The Importance of a Safe and Inclusive Work Environment

Creating a safe and inclusive work environment for autistic adults is essential for their success and wellbeing in the workplace. This can include:

Improving job performance

Increasing job satisfaction

Reducing stress and anxiety

Improving overall wellbeing

Best Practices for Creating a Safe and Inclusive Work Environment

There are many strategies that can be used to create a safe and inclusive work environment for autistic adults. Some best practices include:

Providing accommodations and modifications to support their needs

Providing clear and straightforward communication

Offering training and resources for coworkers to understand and support individuals with autism

Encouraging a culture of respect, understanding, and inclusiveness

The Role of Employers and Coworkers

Employers and coworkers play a crucial role in creating a safe and inclusive work environment for autistic adults. By being aware of the needs of individuals with autism and making appropriate accommodations and modifications, employers and coworkers can help to create a supportive and inclusive work environment.

This may include providing accommodations such as flexible schedules or quiet workspaces, and taking steps to ensure that communication is clear and easy to understand. Additionally, employers and coworkers can support individuals with autism by being understanding and patient, and by avoiding behavior that may cause stress or anxiety.

Addressing Challenges and Barriers

Creating a safe and inclusive work environment for autistic adults can involve addressing challenges and barriers that may arise. This may include:

Addressing negative attitudes and stereotypes

Overcoming communication barriers

Dealing with sensory sensitivities

Managing unpredictable or sudden changes in the workplace

Conclusion

In conclusion, creating a safe and inclusive work environment for autistic adults is essential for their success and wellbeing in the workplace. By understanding their unique needs and challenges, and by taking steps to create a supportive and inclusive work environment, employers and coworkers can help individuals with autism to thrive and succeed in their careers.

Introduction to Encouraging a Positive and Respectful Workplace Culture for Autistic Adults

Autistic adults face unique challenges in the workplace, and it is essential to create a positive and respectful workplace culture that supports and accommodates their needs. This ebook will explore the importance of encouraging a positive and respectful workplace culture for autistic adults, and will provide practical tips and strategies for doing so.

Understanding the Needs of Autistic Adults in the Workplace

Before encouraging a positive and respectful workplace culture for autistic adults, it is important to understand their unique needs and challenges. Some common difficulties faced by autistic individuals in the workplace include social and communication difficulties, sensory sensitivities, and difficulty with change and unpredictability.

The Importance of a Positive and Respectful Workplace Culture

Encouraging a positive and respectful workplace culture for autistic adults is essential for their success and wellbeing in the workplace. This can include:

Improving job performance

Increasing job satisfaction

Reducing stress and anxiety

Improving overall wellbeing

Best Practices for Encouraging a Positive and Respectful Workplace Culture

There are many strategies that can be used to encourage a positive and respectful workplace culture for autistic adults. Some best practices include:

Providing accommodations and modifications to support their needs

Providing clear and straightforward communication

Offering training and resources for coworkers to understand and support individuals with autism

Encouraging open and respectful communication between all employees

Celebrating and promoting diversity and inclusiveness

The Role of Employers and Coworkers

Employers and coworkers play a crucial role in encouraging a positive and respectful workplace culture for autistic adults. By being aware of the needs of individuals with autism and making appropriate accommodations and modifications, employers and coworkers can help to create a supportive and inclusive work environment.

This may include providing accommodations such as flexible schedules or quiet workspaces, and taking steps to ensure that communication is clear and easy to understand. Additionally, employers and coworkers can support individuals with autism by being understanding and patient, and by avoiding behavior that may cause stress or anxiety.

Addressing Challenges and Barriers

Encouraging a positive and respectful workplace culture for autistic adults can involve addressing challenges and barriers that may arise. This may include:

Addressing negative attitudes and stereotypes

Overcoming communication barriers

Dealing with sensory sensitivities

Managing unpredictable or sudden changes in the workplace

Conclusion

In conclusion, encouraging a positive and respectful workplace culture for autistic adults is essential for their success and wellbeing in the workplace. By understanding their unique needs and challenges, and by taking steps to create a supportive and inclusive work environment, employers and coworkers can help individuals with autism to thrive and succeed in their careers.

5 ACCOMMODATING ABILITIES: MAKING WORKPLACE ADJUSTMENTS FOR AUTISTIC ADULTS

Autism, or Autism Spectrum Disorder (ASD), is a neurodevelopmental condition that affects an individual's ability to communicate and interact with others. Autistic individuals often experience difficulties in navigating social and communication interactions, and this can also extend to the workplace. One area of particular concern for autistic adults is the physical environment of the workplace, which can have a significant impact on their sensory sensitivities. In this ebook, we will explore the importance of adapting the physical environment of the workplace to meet the sensory needs of autistic adults.

Understanding Sensory Sensitivities in Autistic Adults

Sensory sensitivities are a common aspect of autism, and individuals with autism can experience heightened or decreased sensitivity to stimuli in the environment. For example, some autistic individuals may be particularly sensitive to loud noises, bright lights, strong smells, or certain textures. These sensitivities can be overwhelming and make it difficult for them to focus on work tasks. It is important for employers to understand and acknowledge these sensitivities and to make reasonable accommodations to accommodate their needs.

The Impact of Sensory Sensitivities on Employment

Sensory sensitivities can have a significant impact on an autistic individual's ability to succeed in the workplace. For example, if an employee is sensitive to bright lights, it can be difficult for them to concentrate on tasks, which can negatively impact their productivity. If an employee is sensitive to loud noises, it can be difficult for them to maintain focus, leading to errors or mistakes. These difficulties can result in increased stress and anxiety for the employee, which can negatively impact their mental health and well-being.

Environmental Considerations for Autistic Adults in the Workplace

Employers can take several steps to help create a sensory-friendly workplace for autistic employees. This can include reducing noise levels, using soft lighting, and limiting strong odors. Additionally, employers can provide a quiet space for employees to retreat to if they become overwhelmed. Providing flexible work arrangements, such as the ability to work from home or in a quiet location, can also be beneficial.

Adapting the Physical Environment

There are many ways in which employers can adapt the physical environment of the workplace to meet the sensory needs of autistic employees. For example, employers can install soundproofing materials, such as sound-absorbing panels, to reduce noise levels. They can also install adjustable lighting, such as dimmer switches, to allow employees to control the brightness of their work environment. Additionally, employers can provide sensory-friendly furniture and equipment, such as adjustable chairs and ergonomic keyboards, to help minimize discomfort and improve focus.

Working with Autistic Adults to Identify Needs

It is important for employers to work closely with their autistic employees to identify their specific sensory needs and preferences. For example, an employee may prefer a quiet workspace with low lighting, while another employee may prefer a bright and bustling environment. Employers can work with their employees to create an individualized plan that meets their specific needs and helps them be successful in their role.

Supporting Autistic Employees

Supporting autistic employees in the workplace requires a proactive and inclusive approach. This can include providing ongoing training and education for managers and coworkers on how to support autistic individuals, and developing policies and procedures that ensure autistic employees are treated fairly and respectfully. Additionally, employers can provide resources, such as counseling or support groups, to help employees manage stress and anxiety related to their work environment.

Autistic adults often face unique challenges in the workplace, including difficulties with change, unpredictability, and navigating social and communication norms. One area where support can be particularly beneficial is in the provision of flexible scheduling and breaks. By understanding the needs of autistic individuals and making reasonable accommodations, employers can create a more inclusive and supportive work environment that benefits both the individual and the organization as a whole.

The Importance of Flexible Scheduling and Breaks for Autistic Adults

For many autistic individuals, a rigid,

structured schedule is important for maintaining stability and reducing anxiety. In the workplace, this can mean that rigid work hours or inflexible break times can cause undue stress and impact performance. Providing flexible scheduling options, such as adjusting work hours to better align with the individual's schedule or allowing for more frequent breaks, can help to reduce stress and increase productivity.

Flexible scheduling can also benefit those with sensory sensitivities, who may need to take additional breaks throughout the day to manage sensory overload. In addition, it can provide much-needed respite for those who find social interaction in the workplace challenging, allowing them to recharge and be more engaged and productive when they return to work.

Creating a Culture of Support

Incorporating flexible scheduling and breaks

into the workplace can be a challenge, but it is essential to create an inclusive and supportive work environment for autistic individuals. Employers and coworkers can play an important role in promoting this culture by valuing the unique strengths and abilities of autistic individuals and recognizing the importance of accommodations in supporting their success.

In order to effectively implement flexible scheduling and breaks, it is important to engage in open and respectful communication with the individual and their team. This can include discussing their needs, exploring potential solutions, and working together to find a mutually beneficial solution that meets the needs of both the individual and the organization.

Practical Strategies for Implementing Flexible Scheduling and Breaks

Open Communication: Encourage open and

honest communication with the individual to understand their specific needs and preferences.

Collaboration: Work with the individual and their team to identify and implement flexible scheduling options that meet the needs of all parties.

Accommodations: Provide accommodations, such as flexible work hours or additional breaks, to support the individual's well-being and performance.

Sensory-Friendly Spaces: Create sensory-friendly spaces where the individual can take breaks or retreat when they need a moment of respite.

Clear Policies: Develop clear policies around flexible scheduling and breaks to ensure consistency and fairness for all employees.

Supportive Supervision: Provide ongoing support and guidance from supervisors and coworkers to ensure that the individual feels valued and supported.

Employee Training: Provide training for all employees on the importance of flexible scheduling and breaks for autistic individuals and how to support their success.

Regular Feedback: Encourage regular feedback from the individual to assess the effectiveness of the accommodations and make necessary adjustments.

Recognition and Celebration: Recognize and celebrate the contributions of autistic individuals and the unique value they bring to the workplace.

Continuous Improvement: Continuously evaluate and refine the accommodations provided to ensure they are effective in supporting the individual's success.

Conclusion

Flexible scheduling and breaks can play an

important role in supporting the success of autistic adults in the workplace. By creating a culture of support, engaging in open communication, and implementing practical strategies, employers can provide a safe and inclusive environment where individuals can thrive. By doing so, we can unlock the full potential of autistic individuals and create a more diverse and inclusive workplace for all.

Autism Spectrum Disorder (ASD) is a neurodevelopmental disorder that affects social interaction, communication, and behavior. Individuals with autism may face a range of challenges in the workplace, including difficulties with social interactions, change and unpredictability, and attention to detail. One of the biggest challenges that autistic adults face in the workplace is a lack of clear job expectations and instructions. This can lead to confusion, frustration, and stress, which can negatively impact job performance.

In this ebook, we will explore the importance of providing clear and concise job expectations and instructions for autistic adults on the job. We will discuss why clear communication and structure are crucial for the success of autistic individuals in the workplace and provide practical strategies that employers and coworkers can use to support autistic individuals in this regard.

Why Clear Communication and Structure are Important

Autistic individuals often thrive in environments that are structured, predictable, and consistent. Clear expectations and instructions can help reduce anxiety, increase understanding, and promote confidence. When autistic individuals have a clear understanding of what is expected of them in their job, they are more likely to be successful and feel valued in their workplace.

Additionally, clear communication and structure can help eliminate confusion and misunderstandings, reducing the risk of miscommunication or mistakes. This can lead to a more positive and productive work environment, benefiting both the individual with autism and the company as a whole.

Practical Strategies for Providing Clear Expectations and Instructions

Use Visual Supports: Autistic individuals often respond well to visual aids, such as diagrams, flowcharts, and checklists. Using visual aids to outline job expectations and instructions can make the information easier to understand and retain.

Break Tasks into Steps: Breaking tasks down into smaller, manageable steps can make the information easier to understand and follow. This can also help the individual with autism see the progression of their work, increasing motivation and productivity.

Provide Written Instructions: Written instructions can be especially helpful for autistic individuals, as they can refer back to them as needed. Written instructions should be clear, concise, and detailed, using simple language whenever possible.

Use Demonstrations: Demonstrations can be a helpful tool for providing instruction and demonstrating expectations. This can help the individual with autism understand the task better and reduce the risk of misinterpretation.

Encourage Questions: Encouraging questions can help the individual with autism understand their job expectations and responsibilities better. It can also provide an opportunity for the individual to clarify any misunderstandings or confusion.

Provide Regular Feedback: Regular

feedback can help the individual with autism understand their progress and areas for improvement. Feedback should be clear, concise, and constructive, focusing on specific behaviors and actions.

Promote Collaboration: Collaborating with coworkers can help the individual with autism understand their job expectations and responsibilities better. It can also provide an opportunity for the individual to ask for clarification or support.

Foster a Positive Work Culture: A positive and supportive work culture can help the individual with autism feel valued and confident in their job. This can lead to increased job satisfaction, motivation, and performance.

Provide Ongoing Support: Ongoing support and guidance can help the individual with autism understand their job expectations and responsibilities better. This can also provide an opportunity for the individual to receive feedback, ask for clarification, and receive support as needed.

Be Flexible: Autistic individuals may need extra time, support, or modifications to perform their job effectively. Employers and coworkers should be flexible and willing to accommodate the needs of the individual with autism to promote success in the workplace.

Introduction

Autism, also known as Autism Spectrum Disorder (ASD), is a neurodevelopmental disorder that affects an individual's ability to communicate and interact socially. Despite the challenges they face in these areas, many autistic adults are capable of holding down a job and making meaningful contributions to the workforce. However, they often face unique difficulties in the workplace that can make it difficult for them to thrive.

One such area of difficulty for autistic adults is social and communication skills in the workplace. Navigating social situations and understanding unwritten workplace norms can be a major challenge for individuals with autism. Additionally, sensory sensitivities and an aversion to change can also impact their experience on the job.

In this ebook, we will explore the social and communication difficulties faced by autistic adults in the workplace and discuss practical solutions to support their success on the job.

Understanding Social and Communication Difficulties in the Workplace

For many individuals with autism, social and communication difficulties are a major challenge in the workplace. Navigating social cues, understanding sarcasm and humor, and participating in group conversations can all be difficult for those with autism. Additionally, they may have trouble expressing themselves clearly, leading to misunderstandings and miscommunications.

Creating a Supportive Work Environment

One of the key ways to support autistic adults in the workplace is to create a supportive work environment. This includes providing clear and concise job expectations, allowing for flexible scheduling and breaks, and making accommodations for sensory sensitivities. Employers can also provide training for coworkers to understand and support their autistic coworkers.

Supporting Social and Communication Needs

There are several ways to support the social and communication needs of autistic adults in the workplace. Providing visual aids, such as schedules and lists, can help with clarity and understanding. Allowing for quiet spaces for breaks and time to decompress can also help mitigate sensory sensitivities. Additionally, having open lines of communication and regularly checking in with autistic employees can help ensure their needs are being met.

Providing Clear and Concise Job Expectations

Autistic individuals often thrive in structured environments with clear expectations. Employers can support their success by providing clear job instructions and expectations. This can include written instructions, demonstration of tasks, and clear guidelines for success in the role.

Adapting the Physical Environment

The physical environment of the workplace can have a significant impact on the well-being of autistic individuals. Providing accommodations such as noise-cancelling headphones, adjustable lighting, and private spaces can help mitigate sensory sensitivities. Employers can also consider making modifications to the physical space to create a more autism-friendly environment.

Encouraging Positive and Respectful Workplace Culture

A positive and respectful workplace culture can have a significant impact on the success of autistic individuals on the job. Employers can encourage this by promoting inclusivity, understanding, and respect for all employees. This can include regular trainings on autism and sensitivity to different communication styles.

Implementing Flexible Scheduling and Breaks

Autistic individuals may have unique needs when it comes to scheduling and breaks. Allowing for flexible schedules and breaks can help mitigate the effects of sensory sensitivities and reduce stress levels. Employers can also consider offering quiet spaces for breaks and time to decompress.

Supporting Sensory Needs

Sensory sensitivities can have a significant impact on the well-being and success of autistic individuals in the workplace. Employers can support their sensory needs by making accommodations such as adjustable lighting, providing quiet spaces for breaks, and avoiding strong scents and loud noises.

ABOUT THE AUTHOR

Author, autism expert, and trombone player from Huntington, Indiana living in Fort Wayne. Exploring the world through travel and connecting with family - especially my two nieces and my sister. Passionate about social behavior.

Breaking the Mold: Empowering Autistic Adults in the Workplace

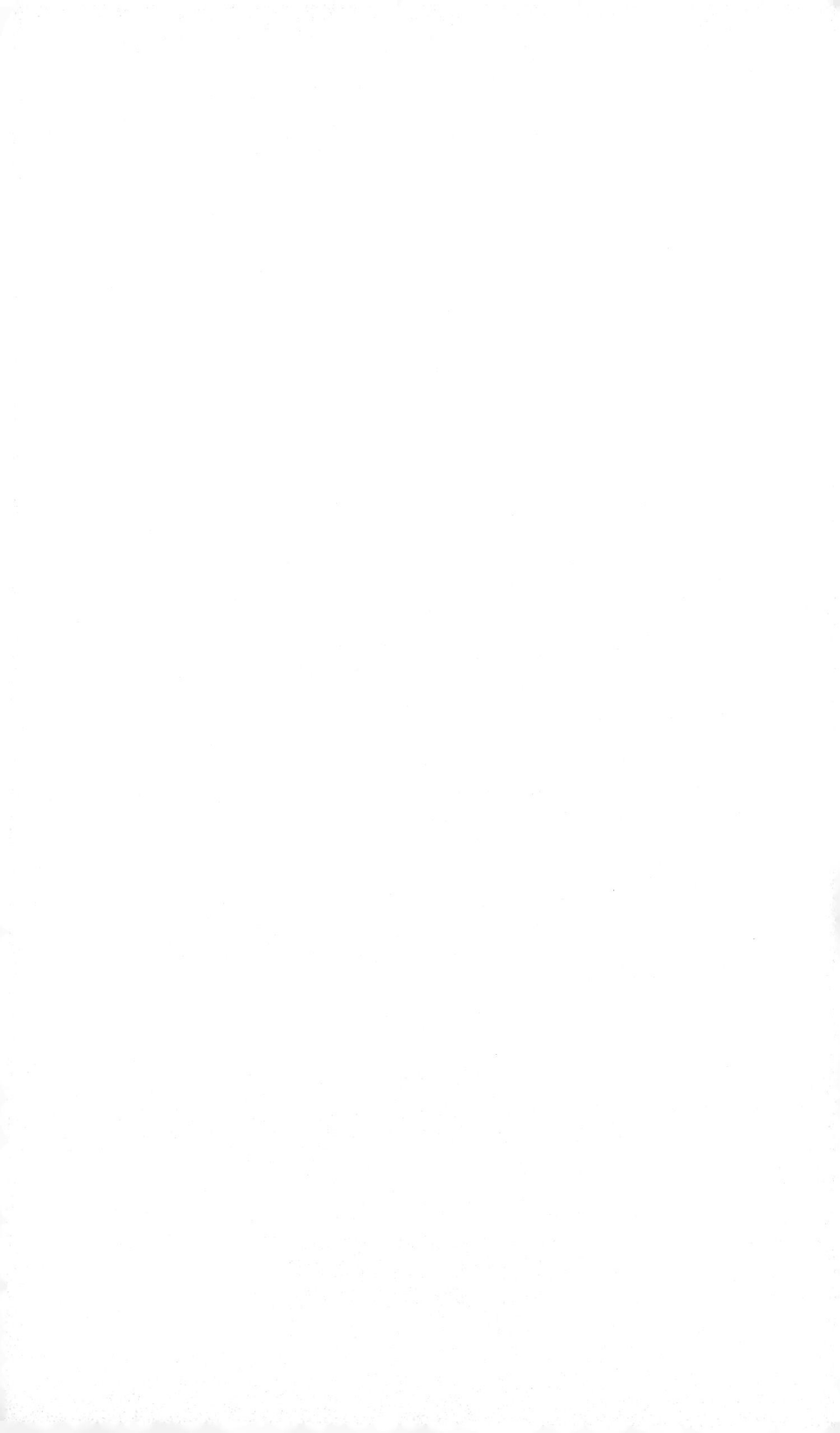

Made in United States
Orlando, FL
05 March 2023